FREE FROM HIGH BLOOD PRESSURE

Holistic Approaches to Lowering High Blood Pressure Naturally"

By Dr Jacob Jabin

BLOOD PRESSURE NATURAL REMEDIES

TABLE OF CONTENTS

BLOOD PRESSURE NATURAL REMEDIES

INTRODUCTION TO HIGH BLOOD PRESSURE

Understanding Blood Pressure

Blood pressure is a vital indicator of overall health and a key factor in assessing cardiovascular well-being. It measures the force exerted by blood against the walls of blood vessels as it circulates through the body. Understanding blood pressure is crucial for maintaining optimal health and preventing the development of cardiovascular diseases. This note aims to provide a comprehensive overview of blood pressure, including its measurement, normal ranges, factors affecting it, and the significance of managing blood pressure levels.

Measurement of Blood Pressure:
Blood pressure is typically measured using a sphygmomanometer, a device consisting of an inflatable cuff, a pressure gauge, and a stethoscope. The measurement involves two values: systolic pressure and diastolic pressure. Systolic pressure represents the force when the heart contracts and pumps blood, while diastolic pressure corresponds to the pressure when the

heart is at rest between beats. Blood pressure is expressed in millimeters of mercury (mmHg), with the systolic value placed over the diastolic value (e.g., 120/80 mmHg).

Normal Blood Pressure Range:
The optimal blood pressure range for adults is typically considered to be around 120/80 mmHg. However, it is important to note that blood pressure can vary among individuals and across different age groups. Blood pressure values above 120/80 mmHg may indicate prehypertension or hypertension, while values below this range may indicate hypotension. Consistently elevated or low blood pressure levels warrant medical attention.

Factors Affecting Blood Pressure:
Several factors can influence blood pressure levels, including:

a. Lifestyle: *Unhealthy habits such as smoking, excessive alcohol consumption, physical inactivity, and a poor diet can contribute to high blood pressure.*

b. Age: *Blood pressure tends to increase with age as blood vessels become less elastic.*

c. Genetics: *Family history of hypertension can increase the risk of developing high blood pressure.*

*d. **Weight:** Excess body weight, especially obesity, can lead to higher blood pressure.*

*e. **Stress:** Chronic stress and anxiety can temporarily raise blood pressure levels.*

*f. **Underlying Medical Conditions:** Conditions such as diabetes, kidney disease, and hormonal disorders can impact blood pressure.*

The Significance of Managing Blood Pressure:
Maintaining healthy blood pressure levels is vital for overall health and well-being. High blood pressure, or hypertension, puts extra strain on the heart and blood vessels, increasing the risk of heart disease, stroke, kidney problems, and other serious health complications. Conversely, low blood pressure, or hypotension, can cause dizziness, fainting, and reduced organ perfusion. Managing blood pressure involves adopting a healthy lifestyle, including regular exercise, a balanced diet, stress management, limiting alcohol consumption, and avoiding smoking. In some cases, medication may be prescribed to control blood pressure effectively.

Risk Factors and Consequences of High Blood Pressure

In the fast-paced world we live in, it is essential to prioritize our health and well-being. Understanding the risk factors and consequences associated with high blood pressure is crucial for taking proactive measures to maintain a healthy lifestyle.

Risk Factors:
High blood pressure, also known as hypertension, can result from a combination of genetic and lifestyle factors. While we cannot control our genetic predisposition, certain lifestyle choices significantly contribute to the development of high blood pressure. Here are some key risk factors:

Unhealthy Diet: *Consuming a diet high in sodium, saturated fats, cholesterol, and processed foods increases the risk of developing hypertension. It is important to prioritize a balanced diet rich in fruits, vegetables, whole grains, lean proteins, and low-fat dairy products.*

Sedentary Lifestyle: *Lack of physical activity weakens the cardiovascular system, leading to an increased likelihood of developing high blood pressure. Regular exercise helps maintain a healthy weight, strengthens the heart, and improves blood circulation.*

Tobacco and Alcohol Consumption: *Smoking and excessive alcohol consumption can raise blood pressure levels and damage blood vessels. Quitting smoking and moderating alcohol intake significantly reduce the risk of hypertension.*

Stress*: Chronic stress can elevate blood pressure temporarily and, over time, contribute to the development of hypertension. Implementing stress management techniques, such as meditation, deep breathing exercises, and engaging in hobbies, can help alleviate stress and promote overall well-being.*

Age and Family History: *As we age, the risk of high blood pressure increases. Additionally, if your close family members have a history of hypertension, you may be more susceptible to developing the condition. Regular blood pressure screenings and adopting a healthy lifestyle are vital in such cases.*

Consequences:
Untreated or uncontrolled high blood pressure can lead to severe complications, affecting various organs and systems within the body. Some of the consequences include:

Cardiovascular Diseases: *Hypertension puts a strain on the heart, increasing the risk of coronary artery disease, heart attack, heart failure, and abnormal heart rhythms. It can also lead to the development of* atherosclerosis, a condition where the arteries become narrowed and hardened.

Stroke: High blood pressure is a leading cause of strokes. It damages blood vessels in the brain, resulting in reduced blood flow, and increases the likelihood of blood clots or hemorrhages.

Kidney Damage: Prolonged hypertension can impair the kidneys' ability to filter waste from the blood properly, leading to kidney disease or kidney failure.

Vision Problems: The tiny blood vessels in the eyes can be damaged by high blood pressure, potentially causing vision loss or retinopathy.

Cognitive Decline: Chronic high blood pressure is associated with an increased risk of cognitive decline, dementia, and Alzheimer's disease.

It is important to note that these risk factors and consequences are not exhaustive, but they underscore the significance of managing high blood pressure effectively.
Remember, small changes in your daily routine can make a significant difference in your overall health. Take care of your well-being today to enjoy a healthier and more fulfilling tomorrow.

LIFESTYLE MODIFICATIONS FOR MANAGING HIGH BLOOD PRESSURE

Dietary Changes

High blood pressure, also known as hypertension, is a chronic medical condition that affects a significant portion of the global population. It is a major risk factor for various cardiovascular diseases, including heart attack and stroke. While medical interventions such as medication may be necessary, lifestyle modifications, including dietary changes, play a crucial role in managing and controlling high blood pressure. This note focuses on the dietary changes that individuals can adopt to help manage their blood pressure levels effectively.

Reduce Sodium Intake:

Excessive sodium consumption is strongly associated with high blood pressure. Limiting the intake of sodium is important for managing hypertension. Individuals should aim to consume no more than 2,300 milligrams (mg) of sodium per day, and further reduce it to 1,500 mg or less if they have hypertension or are at high risk. To achieve this, it is essential to read food labels, choose low-sodium options, avoid processed and fast foods, and minimize the use of salt in cooking.

Increase Potassium-Rich Foods:
Potassium intake helps counteract the effects of sodium on blood pressure. Including potassium-rich foods in the diet can help lower blood pressure levels. Some excellent sources of potassium include fruits (such as bananas, oranges, and avocados), vegetables (like spinach, sweet potatoes, and tomatoes), legumes, nuts, and seeds.

Emphasize a Balanced Diet:
Following a balanced diet, such as the Dietary Approaches to Stop Hypertension (DASH) eating plan, can be beneficial in managing high blood pressure. The DASH diet encourages the consumption of fruits, vegetables, whole grains, lean proteins (such as fish, poultry, and beans), and low-fat dairy products. It also promotes limiting saturated and trans fats, cholesterol, processed foods, sugary beverages, and excessive alcohol consumption.

Adopt a Mediterranean-style Diet:
The Mediterranean diet, rich in fruits, vegetables, whole grains, legumes, lean proteins (including fish and poultry), and healthy fats (such as olive oil and nuts), has been associated with numerous health benefits, including reduced blood pressure. This dietary pattern also emphasizes reducing sodium intake and limiting processed foods, red meat, and sugary desserts.

Monitor Portion Sizes and Caloric Intake:

Weight management plays a significant role in blood pressure control. Monitoring portion sizes and maintaining a healthy weight is crucial. Overeating and consuming excess calories can contribute to weight gain and elevated blood pressure. It is advisable to practice mindful eating, control portion sizes, and pay attention to the body's hunger and satiety cues.

Limit Alcohol Consumption:
Excessive alcohol intake can raise blood pressure. It is advisable to limit alcohol consumption to moderate levels, which means up to one drink per day for women and up to two drinks per day for men. However, it is important to note that individuals with hypertension or other health conditions may need to avoid alcohol altogether.

DASH (Dietary Approaches to Stop Hypertension) Diet

High blood pressure, or hypertension, is a prevalent health condition affecting millions of individuals worldwide. To effectively manage and reduce blood pressure levels, lifestyle modifications play a crucial role. Among these modifications, the Dietary Approaches to Stop Hypertension (DASH) diet has gained significant recognition as a scientifically proven approach. Developed by the National Heart, Lung, and Blood Institute (NHLBI), the DASH diet offers a balanced and nutritious eating plan that emphasizes key food groups while limiting sodium intake. This note explores the principles, benefits, and key components of the DASH diet as an effective strategy for managing high blood pressure.

Principles of the DASH Diet:

Emphasis on Fruits and Vegetables: *The DASH diet encourages the consumption of a variety of fruits and vegetables, which are rich in essential nutrients, fiber, and antioxidants. These components contribute to overall heart health and help control blood pressure.*

Whole Grains and Lean Protein: *The DASH diet emphasizes whole grains, such as brown rice and whole* wheat bread, as well as lean protein sources like poultry, fish, and legumes. These foods are low in saturated fats and cholesterol, reducing the risk of cardiovascular disease.

Low-Fat Dairy Products: Low-fat or fat-free dairy products, such as skim milk and yogurt, are included in the DASH diet. They provide essential nutrients like calcium and potassium, which help regulate blood pressure.

Limited Sodium Intake: The DASH diet restricts sodium intake to 2,300 milligrams (mg) per day, or even lower (1,500 mg per day) for individuals with higher blood pressure or other risk factors. Reducing sodium intake helps prevent fluid retention and lower blood pressure.

Moderation in Added Sugars and Red Meat: The DASH diet advises moderate consumption of added sugars, sugary beverages, and red meat. Limiting these foods helps manage weight and reduce the risk of cardiovascular complications.

Benefits of the DASH Diet:

Blood Pressure Management: The DASH diet's primary objective is to lower blood pressure levels. Studies have consistently shown that adopting the DASH eating plan can lead to significant reductions in both systolic and diastolic blood pressure.

Cardiovascular Health: *The DASH diet promotes heart health by reducing the risk of cardiovascular diseases, including heart attacks, strokes, and heart failure. Its emphasis on nutrient-rich foods and limited intake of unhealthy fats supports overall cardiovascular well-being.*

Weight Management: *The DASH diet's emphasis on whole grains, fruits, vegetables, and lean proteins, coupled with limited saturated fats and added sugars, aids in weight management. Maintaining a healthy weight contributes to better blood pressure control.*

Nutritional Adequacy: *The DASH diet provides a well-balanced eating plan that supplies essential nutrients, including potassium, magnesium, calcium, and fiber. These nutrients have beneficial effects on blood pressure regulation and overall health.*

Incorporating the DASH Diet into Lifestyle Modifications:

Gradual Transition: *Start by gradually implementing the DASH diet principles into your eating habits, allowing your taste buds and body to adapt to the changes.*

Meal Planning: *Plan your meals in advance to ensure you have DASH-friendly ingredients readily available.*

This helps you make healthier food choices and reduces the reliance on processed or high-sodium foods.

Read Food Labels: *Pay attention to nutrition labels, particularly the sodium content, when purchasing packaged foods. Opt for lower-sodium alternatives whenever possible.*

Home Cooking: *Preparing meals at home allows you to have control over the ingredients and cooking methods, ensuring your meals align with the DASH diet principles.*

Consultation with a Healthcare Professional: *If you have existing health conditions or take medications, consult with a healthcare professional or a registered dietitian before making significant dietary changes.*

The DASH diet offers a comprehensive and scientifically backed dietary approach for managing high blood pressure. By emphasizing nutrient-rich foods, reducing sodium intake, and promoting overall healthy eating habits, the DASH diet contributes to blood pressure control, cardiovascular health, and weight management. Incorporating the DASH diet into lifestyle modifications can yield long-term benefits and support overall well-being. Remember to consult with healthcare professionals for personalized guidance when making significant dietary changes.

Sodium Restriction

If you have been diagnosed with high blood pressure (hypertension), one crucial aspect of your lifestyle modification involves sodium restriction. Sodium, commonly found in table salt and many processed foods, can contribute to elevated blood pressure levels. Adopting a diet low in sodium can play a significant role in managing your condition and reducing the risk of associated health complications.

Here are some key points to consider regarding sodium restriction when dealing with high blood pressure:

Sodium's Impact on Blood Pressure: *Sodium plays a role in regulating the balance of fluids in your body. When you consume excessive sodium, it retains water, causing increased fluid volume in your bloodstream. The extra fluid puts more pressure on your blood vessels, leading to elevated blood pressure levels.*

Recommended Sodium Intake: *The American Heart Association (AHA) suggests limiting daily sodium intake to 1,500-2,300 milligrams (mg) for most individuals, especially those with hypertension. However, consult with your healthcare provider to determine the appropriate sodium restriction that suits your specific health needs.*

Reading Food Labels: *It is essential to carefully read and understand food labels to identify sodium content in* various products. Pay attention to the "sodium" or "salt" content per serving size. Be mindful that sodium is not only present in obvious sources like table salt but also in processed foods such as canned soups, condiments, deli meats, and fast food items.

Lowering Sodium in Your Diet: Here are some practical strategies to reduce sodium intake:

Cook at home: Preparing meals yourself from scratch allows you to control the amount of sodium added to your dishes.

Choose fresh foods: Opt for fresh fruits, vegetables, and whole grains, which are naturally low in sodium.

Limit processed foods: Minimize your consumption of processed and packaged foods, as they often contain high levels of sodium.

Use herbs and spices: Enhance the flavor of your meals with herbs, spices, and other salt-free seasonings to reduce reliance on salt for taste.

Be cautious eating out: When dining out, request for dishes to be prepared with less salt or choose options labeled as low-sodium.

Monitoring Hidden Sodium: Some food items may not taste salty but can still have high sodium content. Examples include cheese, bread, certain cereals, and *even some medications. It's advisable to consult your healthcare provider or a registered dietitian for guidance on identifying hidden sources of sodium in your diet.*

Remember, while sodium restriction is essential for managing high blood pressure, it is just one component of an overall healthy lifestyle.

Potassium-Rich Foods

High blood pressure, or hypertension, is a common condition that can significantly impact your health if left unmanaged. Lifestyle modifications play a crucial role in managing high blood pressure, and one important aspect is incorporating a diet rich in potassium. Potassium is an essential mineral that helps regulate blood pressure levels by counteracting the effects of sodium.

Including potassium-rich foods in your diet can be an effective way to lower blood pressure naturally. Here are some key points about potassium-rich foods and their benefits:

Role of Potassium: *Potassium helps maintain a healthy blood pressure level by promoting the excretion of excess sodium through urine. It also helps relax the walls of blood vessels, reducing strain on the cardiovascular system.*

Recommended Daily Intake: *The recommended daily intake of potassium for adults is around 2,500 to 3,000 milligrams (mg). However, this may vary depending on individual health conditions, so it's best to consult with a healthcare professional for personalized advice.*

Potassium-Rich Foods: *Incorporate the following potassium-rich foods into your diet:*

Fruits: *Bananas, oranges, apricots, kiwi, avocados, and melons (such as cantaloupe and honeydew) are excellent sources of potassium.*

Vegetables: *Leafy greens like spinach and kale, tomatoes, sweet potatoes, potatoes, broccoli, and Brussels sprouts are rich in potassium.*

Legumes: *Beans (such as kidney beans, black beans, and pinto beans), lentils, and peas are all high in potassium.*

Dairy and Dairy Alternatives: *Low-fat milk, yogurt, and soy milk can be good sources of potassium. Be mindful of the added sugars in some flavored dairy products.*

Nuts and Seeds: *Almonds, pistachios, peanuts, and sunflower seeds are all potassium-rich options for snacking.*

Dietary Considerations: *When increasing your potassium intake, it's important to maintain a balanced diet and consider overall nutritional needs. If you have any underlying health conditions or are taking medications, consult with a healthcare professional to ensure your dietary changes align with your specific needs.*

Other Lifestyle Modifications: *While focusing on a potassium-rich diet, it's also essential to adopt other lifestyle modifications for managing high blood pressure.*

These include reducing sodium intake, maintaining a healthy weight, engaging in regular physical activity, limiting alcohol consumption, managing stress levels, and quitting smoking.

By incorporating potassium-rich foods into your diet as part of a holistic approach to managing high blood pressure, you can contribute to better cardiovascular health and overall well-being.

Magnesium and Calcium Intake

Magnesium is an important mineral that plays a very good role in maintaining cardiovascular health. It helps regulate blood pressure by relaxing the blood vessels, which reduces resistance to blood flow and lowers overall blood pressure. Additionally, magnesium helps to balance electrolytes, including potassium and sodium, which are important for maintaining proper blood pressure levels.

Increasing magnesium intake can be achieved through dietary sources such as green leafy vegetables, whole grains, nuts, seeds, and legumes. Alternatively, magnesium supplements may be considered under the guidance of a healthcare professional. The recommended daily allowance for magnesium varies depending on age and sex, but adults generally require around 320-420 mg per day.

Calcium is another mineral that plays a crucial role in maintaining healthy blood pressure levels. It is involved in regulating muscle contraction, including the muscles in the blood vessels. Adequate calcium intake can help relax the blood vessels, leading to lower blood pressure.

Dietary sources of calcium include dairy products, leafy greens, fortified cereals, and certain types of fish like salmon and sardines. Calcium supplements may also be recommended if dietary intake is insufficient. However, it is important to note that excessive calcium intake from supplements may have adverse effects, so it is best to consult with a healthcare professional before starting any supplementation. The daily intake of calcium recommended for adults ranges from 1000-1300 mg.

It's important to emphasize that while magnesium and calcium intake can contribute to the management of high blood pressure, they are just one aspect of a comprehensive lifestyle approach. Other modifications, such as adopting a balanced diet rich in fruits, vegetables, whole grains, and lean proteins, reducing sodium intake, engaging in regular physical activity, managing stress levels, and maintaining a healthy weight, are all important for blood pressure control.

Regular Exercise

Engaging in regular physical activity not only helps lower blood pressure but also contributes to overall cardiovascular health and well-being. This note highlights the importance of regular exercise as a lifestyle modification for managing high blood pressure.

Benefits of Regular Exercise:

Blood Pressure Control: *Regular exercise has been shown to reduce blood pressure levels, both systolic* and diastolic. It helps strengthen the heart, making it more efficient at pumping blood and reducing the pressure on the arteries.

Weight Management: Exercise aids in weight loss and weight maintenance, which is vital for managing high blood pressure. Maintaining a healthy weight can help reduce the strain on the cardiovascular system and decrease blood pressure.

Improved Cardiovascular Health: Engaging in aerobic activities such as brisk walking, jogging, cycling, or swimming enhances cardiovascular fitness. Regular exercise helps to improve heart function, increase the elasticity of blood vessels, and promote optimal blood flow, all of which contribute to lower blood pressure.

Stress Reduction: Exercise is an excellent stress reliever. Physical activity stimulates the production of endorphins, which are natural mood elevators. Regular exercise helps combat stress and anxiety, both of which can contribute to high blood pressure.

Enhanced Insulin Sensitivity: Regular exercise improves insulin sensitivity, allowing the body to use glucose more effectively. This benefit is particularly important for individuals with high blood pressure, as they often have underlying insulin resistance or type 2 diabetes.

Incorporating Exercise into Daily Routine:

Consult a Healthcare Professional: *Before starting any exercise program, it is advisable to consult a healthcare professional, especially if you have pre-existing health conditions. They can provide guidance tailored to your specific needs and suggest appropriate exercises.*

Choose Activities You Enjoy: *Engaging in physical activities that you enjoy increases the likelihood of long-term adherence. It could be walking, swimming, dancing, cycling, or participating in a team sport. Experiment with different activities to find what suits your interests and fits into your lifestyle.*

Gradual Progression: *Start slowly and gradually increase the duration and intensity of your exercise sessions. Aim for at least 150 minutes of moderate-intensity aerobic activity or 75 minutes of vigorous-intensity aerobic activity per week, spread across several days.*

Stay Consistent: *Consistency is key. Make exercise a habitual thing by scheduling it into your daily routine. Find ways to stay motivated, such as exercising with a friend or using fitness apps to track your progress.*

Monitor Blood Pressure: *Regularly monitor your blood pressure to track the effects of exercise on your hypertension. It will help you and your healthcare* *provider assess the effectiveness of your exercise program and make any necessary adjustments.*

Regular exercise is a valuable lifestyle modification for managing high blood pressure. By incorporating physical activity into your daily routine, you can lower blood pressure, improve cardiovascular health, manage weight, reduce stress, and enhance overall well-being.

Aerobic Exercises

Aerobic exercises, in particular, are highly beneficial for individuals with high blood pressure. These exercises involve rhythmic and continuous movements that increase heart rate and oxygen intake. Here are some key points about aerobic exercises in the context of managing high blood pressure:

Benefits of Aerobic Exercises: *Engaging in regular aerobic exercises has numerous advantages for individuals with high blood pressure. These exercises improve cardiovascular fitness, enhance blood circulation, strengthen the heart muscle, and help maintain a healthy weight. They also contribute to stress reduction and promote overall well-being.*

Recommended Types of Aerobic Exercises: *There are various forms of aerobic exercises that can be incorporated into a hypertension management plan. Some popular options include brisk walking, jogging, cycling, swimming, dancing, and aerobic classes. It's important to choose activities that you like and enjoy and can sustain over time.*

Duration and Frequency: *The American Heart Association recommends engaging in at least 150 minutes of moderate-intensity aerobic exercise or 75 minutes of vigorous-intensity aerobic exercise each week. Ideally, individuals with high blood pressure should aim for 30 minutes of exercise on most days of* *the week. However, even shorter sessions of aerobic activity can be beneficial if done consistently.*

Safety Considerations: *Before starting any exercise program, it's essential to consult with a healthcare professional, especially if you have existing health conditions. This ensures that the chosen exercises are safe and appropriate for your individual situation. Additionally, it's important to start gradually and increase intensity and duration over time.*

Monitoring Intensity: *Monitoring the intensity of aerobic exercises is crucial for individuals with high blood pressure. The perceived exertion scale or target heart rate can be used to assess the intensity level. Generally, a moderate-intensity exercise should make you slightly breathless but still able to carry on a conversation.*

Complementary Lifestyle Modifications: *Aerobic exercises work best when combined with other lifestyle modifications for managing high blood pressure. These include adopting a healthy diet (such as the DASH diet), reducing sodium intake, quitting smoking, limiting alcohol consumption, and managing stress through relaxation techniques or mindfulness practices.*

Remember, consistency is key when it comes to aerobic exercises and managing high blood pressure. Incorporating regular physical activity into your routine, along with other lifestyle modifications, can have a positive impact on your blood pressure levels and overall health.

Strength Training

Alongside a healthy diet, regular physical activity is a key component of a hypertension management plan. While aerobic exercise is often emphasized, strength training also offers numerous benefits for individuals with high blood pressure.

Strength training, also known as resistance training or weightlifting, involves exercises that target and strengthen muscles through the use of resistance. These exercises can include weightlifting, resistance band exercises, bodyweight exercises, or using weight machines. Here are some important points to consider regarding strength training and its role in managing high blood pressure:

Blood Pressure Reduction: Engaging in regular strength training has been shown to help lower blood pressure levels. Studies have shown that strength training can cause a decrease in the systolic (top number) and diastolic (bottom number) blood pressure readings. By enhancing overall cardiovascular fitness and improving blood flow, strength training contributes to reduced blood pressure over time.

Muscle Development: Strength training helps in building and toning muscles, which has a positive impact on blood pressure regulation. As muscles become stronger, they become more efficient at utilizing oxygen and nutrients. This efficiency can enhance the *body's overall cardiovascular function, leading to better blood pressure control.*

Weight Management: *Strength training can aid in weight management, another important aspect of hypertension control. Regular strength training exercises increase muscle mass and metabolism, which helps burn more calories even at rest. When combined with a balanced diet, strength training can contribute to weight loss or maintenance, thus reducing the risk of high blood pressure.*

Improved Insulin Sensitivity: *Strength training has been associated with improved insulin sensitivity, meaning the body becomes more efficient at utilizing glucose from the bloodstream. By enhancing insulin sensitivity, strength training helps maintain stable blood sugar levels, which is important for individuals with high blood pressure as diabetes and hypertension often coexist.*

Mental Health Benefits: *Engaging in regular strength training not only improves physical health but also has positive effects on mental well-being. Exercise, including strength training, releases endorphins, which are natural mood-enhancing chemicals. It helps reduce stress, anxiety, and depression, which can have an indirect impact on blood pressure control.*

Before starting a strength training program, it is essential to consult with a healthcare professional, especially if you have any pre-existing health conditions or concerns. They can provide guidance on appropriate exercises, intensity, and safety precautions based on your individual circumstances.

Incorporating strength training into a lifestyle modification plan for managing high blood pressure offers several advantages. It helps lower blood pressure, promotes muscle development, assists with weight management, improves insulin sensitivity, and enhances mental well-being. By incorporating strength training alongside other healthy habits, individuals can take proactive steps toward controlling their blood pressure and improving overall cardiovascular health.

Yoga and Meditation

Among the various lifestyle changes, incorporating yoga and meditation practices can be particularly beneficial in managing high blood pressure .

Yoga, an ancient practice originating from India, combines physical postures, controlled breathing, and meditation techniques to promote physical, mental, and emotional well-being. Regular practice of yoga has been shown to reduce blood pressure levels and improve overall cardiovascular health. The various yoga asanas (postures) and pranayama (breathing exercises) help relax the body, reduce stress, and improve blood circulation.

Some specific yoga asanas that are known to be beneficial for managing high blood pressure include:

***Savasana (Corpse Pose):** This posture involves lying flat on your back, arms relaxed by your sides, and focusing on deep, slow breathing. It promotes relaxation, reduces stress, and helps lower blood pressure.*

***Viparita Karani (Legs-Up-the-Wall Pose):** In this pose, you lie on your back with your legs resting against a wall. It encourages relaxation and helps improve blood flow, reducing hypertension.*

"Sukhasana" (Easy Pose) and Padmasana (Lotus Pose): *These seated postures promote calmness, mental clarity, and help regulate blood pressure by reducing stress and anxiety.*

In addition to yoga, meditation is another powerful tool for managing high blood pressure. Meditation involves focusing one's attention and eliminating the stream of thoughts that may be causing stress and anxiety. Regular meditation practice has been found to lower blood pressure, reduce stress hormone levels, and promote relaxation.

Mindfulness meditation, where one focuses on the present moment without judgment, has been particularly effective in managing hypertension. It helps individuals develop an awareness of their body and mind, allowing them to identify and control stress triggers that may contribute to high blood pressure.

Combining yoga and meditation in a regular practice routine can have significant benefits for managing high blood pressure. It is important to note that these practices should be done under the guidance of a qualified instructor, especially if you have any pre-existing health conditions or limitations.

Incorporating yoga and meditation into your lifestyle modifications for managing high blood pressure can be highly beneficial. These practices help reduce stress, promote relaxation, and improve overall cardiovascular health. However, it is essential to consult with your healthcare provider and receive proper guidance to ensure that these practices align with your specific health needs and conditions.

Weight Management

High blood pressure, also known as hypertension, is a common condition that can increase the risk of various health problems, including heart disease and stroke. Lifestyle modifications play a crucial role in managing high blood pressure, and one important aspect is weight management.

Maintaining a healthy weight is vital for managing high blood pressure. Excess weight puts strain on the heart and blood vessels, leading to an increase in blood pressure. Additionally, obesity is often associated with other risk factors such as high cholesterol and diabetes, which can further exacerbate hypertension.

Here are some key points to consider regarding weight management for managing high blood pressure:

Body Mass Index (BMI): *Calculate your BMI, which is a measure of body fat based on your height and weight. A healthy BMI range is typically considered to be between 18.5 and 24.9. If your BMI falls within the overweight or* obese category, losing weight can significantly improve blood pressure levels.

Caloric Intake: Monitor your caloric intake and aim to create a calorie deficit if you need to lose weight. Consuming fewer calories than you burn will promote weight loss. Incorporate a balanced diet rich in fruits, vegetables, whole grains, lean proteins, and low-fat dairy products. Limit the intake of processed foods, sugary snacks, and beverages that are high in added sugars.

Physical Activity: Engage in regular physical activity to support weight management and lower blood pressure. Try to practice at least 150 minutes of moderate-intensity aerobic exercise or 75 minutes of vigorous-intensity exercise every week. Incorporate activities you enjoy, such as walking, swimming, cycling, or dancing, into your routine.

Resistance Training: Include resistance training exercises at least two days a week to build muscle mass and increase metabolism. This can help in burning more calories and promoting weight loss.

Eating less: Reducing the amount of food you eat at a time is very important.
Remember that weight management is a long-term commitment. Gradual, sustainable weight loss is more beneficial and easier to maintain than quick, drastic measures.

Stress Reduction Techniques

Alongside medication and dietary changes, incorporating stress reduction techniques into one's lifestyle can play a crucial role in managing and controlling high blood pressure. Chronic stress can contribute to elevated blood pressure levels, so adopting stress reduction techniques can have a positive impact on overall health. Here are some effective stress reduction techniques that can be helpful in managing high blood pressure:

Relaxation techniques: *Practices such as deep breathing exercises, progressive muscle relaxation, and guided imagery can help promote relaxation, reduce muscle tension, and alleviate stress. These techniques can be easily learned and practiced regularly to induce a state of calm and tranquility.*

Mindfulness meditation: *Mindfulness meditation entails focusing one's attention on the current moment without judgment. It can help in reducing stress, lowering blood pressure, and improving overall well-being. Regular practice of mindfulness meditation can enhance self-awareness and promote a sense of inner peace.*

Physical activity: *Engaging in regular physical exercise not only improves cardiovascular fitness but also helps reduce stress and lower blood pressure. Activities such as walking, jogging, cycling, swimming, or participating in sports can effectively relieve stress and contribute to better blood pressure control.*

Yoga and "Tai Chi": *These mind-body practices combine physical movements, deep breathing, and meditation techniques. Both yoga and Tai Chi have been found to reduce stress, lower blood pressure, and enhance overall relaxation. Incorporating these practices into a daily routine can bring about significant benefits for managing hypertension.*

Social support: *Building a strong support network and fostering positive relationships with family, friends, and community can provide emotional support and reduce stress levels. Sharing concerns and seeking support from loved ones can help alleviate anxiety and promote a sense of well-being.*

Time management and prioritization: *Stress often arises from feeling overwhelmed and having too much on one's plate. Effective time management techniques, such as setting realistic goals, prioritizing tasks, and delegating responsibilities, can help reduce stress levels. By organizing and managing time efficiently, individuals can create a more balanced lifestyle.*

Limiting Alcohol and Tobacco Consumption

High blood pressure, also known as hypertension, is a significant risk factor for cardiovascular diseases and other health complications. Lifestyle modifications play a crucial role in managing and preventing high blood pressure. Among these modifications, limiting alcohol and tobacco consumption can have a significant impact on blood pressure control and overall health.

Effects of Alcohol Consumption on Blood Pressure: *Excessive alcohol consumption can lead to an increase in blood pressure. Regular and heavy drinking raises blood pressure levels and also reduces the effectiveness of hypertension medications. Moreover, alcohol can contribute to weight gain, which further exacerbates hypertension. It is recommended that individuals with high blood pressure limit their alcohol intake to moderate levels or avoid it altogether.*

Recommended Alcohol Consumption: *Mild alcohol consumption is defined as up to one drink a day for women and up to two drinks per day for men. However, it's important to note that even moderate alcohol intake may not be suitable for everyone, especially those with certain medical conditions or those taking specific medications. Consulting with a healthcare professional* *is essential to determine the most appropriate alcohol consumption level for individuals with hypertension.*

Impact of Tobacco Use on Blood Pressure:
Smoking and the use of tobacco products significantly increase the risk of developing high blood pressure. The chemicals in tobacco smoke damage blood vessels, causing them to narrow and harden, leading to elevated blood pressure. Additionally, smoking reduces the oxygen content in the blood, making the heart work harder to deliver oxygen to the body's organs. Quitting smoking and avoiding tobacco products is vital for blood pressure management and overall cardiovascular health.

Benefits of Limiting Alcohol and Tobacco Consumption:

Lowered Blood Pressure: *By reducing or eliminating alcohol and tobacco use, individuals can experience a decrease in blood pressure levels, reducing their risk of heart disease, stroke, and other related complications.*
Enhanced Medication Effectiveness: *Limiting alcohol intake ensures that hypertension medications work more effectively, improving blood pressure control.*
Weight Management: *Alcohol and tobacco use are associated with weight gain and increased visceral fat, which can contribute to hypertension. By reducing or eliminating these habits, individuals can maintain a healthy weight and manage blood pressure more effectively.*

Overall Health Improvement: *Limiting alcohol and tobacco consumption has numerous other health benefits, including reduced risk of various cancers, respiratory diseases, and improved lung function.*

Lifestyle modifications, including limiting alcohol and tobacco consumption, are vital for managing high blood pressure. By adhering to recommended alcohol consumption guidelines and quitting smoking or avoiding tobacco products, individuals can significantly lower their blood pressure levels and reduce the risk of cardiovascular diseases.

Caffeine Intake Moderation

One important aspect of lifestyle modification is moderating caffeine intake.
Caffeine is a stimulant found in various beverages and foods, such as coffee, tea, energy drinks, chocolate, and some medications. It acts by stimulating the central nervous system, which can temporarily raise blood pressure. However, the impact of caffeine on blood pressure can vary from person to person.

Studies have shown that consuming moderate amounts of caffeine, typically defined as 200 to 300 milligrams per day (equivalent to about 1 to 3 cups of coffee), generally does not have a significant long-term effect on blood pressure levels in most individuals. However, people who are more sensitive to the effects of caffeine or have pre-existing hypertension may experience an increase in blood pressure after consuming even small amounts of caffeine.

To moderate caffeine intake for better blood pressure management, individuals with high blood pressure or those aiming to prevent hypertension can consider the following tips:

Know your caffeine sources: *Be aware of the caffeine content in various beverages, foods, and medications. Read labels and choose caffeine-free or low-caffeine alternatives whenever possible.*

Limit coffee and tea consumption: *If you regularly consume coffee or tea, consider reducing your intake or opting for decaffeinated versions. Decaffeinated options can provide a similar flavor without the stimulating effects of caffeine.*

Watch out for hidden caffeine: *Caffeine is present in various products, including soda, energy drinks, chocolate, and some medications. Pay attention to these sources and moderate your consumption accordingly.*

Monitor your body's response: *Everyone reacts differently to caffeine. If you notice that caffeine intake affects your blood pressure or overall well-being, it may be necessary to further reduce or eliminate it from your diet.*

Stay hydrated: *Proper hydration is essential for maintaining healthy blood pressure levels. Opt for water or herbal teas as alternatives to caffeinated beverages to stay hydrated without the additional caffeine.*

Natural Supplements and Herbs

Garlic

Garlic, known for its strong aroma and distinctive taste, has been used for centuries for its medicinal properties. Among its many potential health benefits, garlic has gained attention for its purported ability to help manage high blood pressure, also known as hypertension. While garlic is not a substitute for medical treatment, several studies have explored its potential effects on blood pressure regulation. This short note aims to provide an overview of the topic.

Garlic and Blood Pressure:

Blood Pressure Reduction: *Some studies suggest that garlic may have a modest effect in reducing blood pressure levels. The active compounds in garlic, particularly sulfur-containing compounds like allicin, are believed to promote relaxation of blood vessels and improve blood flow, thereby contributing to blood pressure regulation.*

Vasodilation: *Garlic has been shown to possess vasodilatory properties, which means it may help widen blood vessels, leading to reduced resistance and lower blood pressure. This effect could be attributed to the* release of nitric oxide, a compound involved in vascular relaxation.

Antioxidant Properties: *Garlic contains antioxidants that may protect against oxidative stress and inflammation, both of which can contribute to hypertension. By reducing oxidative damage and inflammation, garlic may help maintain healthy blood vessels and overall cardiovascular health.*

Antiplatelet Activity: *Garlic has been suggested to possess antiplatelet properties, meaning it may inhibit the formation of blood clots. This could be beneficial for individuals with hypertension, as blood clot formation can further narrow blood vessels and increase the risk of complications.*

Usage and Considerations:

Garlic Supplements: *Garlic can be consumed in various forms, including raw cloves, cooked dishes, or as a supplement in the form of capsules or tablets. Garlic supplements are standardized to contain specific amounts of the active compounds, and their usage should be discussed with a healthcare professional.*

Potential Side Effects: *While garlic is generally safe for most people, it can cause digestive discomfort, heartburn, and allergic reactions in some individuals. Garlic may also interact with certain medications, such as blood-thinning drugs, so it's important to consult a* healthcare provider before incorporating it into your routine.

Individual Variation: The effects of garlic on blood pressure can vary from person to person. It is important to note that garlic alone is unlikely to provide significant blood pressure reduction, and its use should be seen as a complementary approach alongside lifestyle modifications and prescribed treatments.

Hawthorn

Hawthorn, scientifically known as Crataegus, is a plant that has been used for centuries in traditional medicine to support cardiovascular health. While it may have some potential benefits for managing certain cardiovascular conditions, such as high blood pressure, it is important to note that it should not replace medical advice or prescribed treatments. Here is a brief overview of how hawthorn may be used in relation to high blood pressure:

Vasodilation: Hawthorn has been suggested to promote vasodilation, which is the widening of blood vessels. This effect may help to reduce blood pressure by easing the flow of blood through the vessels, potentially decreasing resistance.

Antioxidant properties: *Hawthorn contains antioxidants that can help protect blood vessels from damage caused by oxidative stress. By reducing oxidative stress, hawthorn may contribute to maintaining healthy blood pressure levels.*

Improved cardiac function: *Hawthorn has been found to have positive effects on heart function. It may enhance the strength of heart contractions and improve blood circulation, potentially assisting in managing high blood pressure.*

Diuretic effects: *Some research suggests that hawthorn may have mild diuretic properties, meaning it could promote increased urine production. This can aid in reducing fluid retention and potentially help lower blood pressure.*

Fish Oil/Omega-3 Fatty Acids

High blood pressure, or hypertension, is a prevalent medical condition that significantly increases the risk of cardiovascular diseases. Lifestyle modifications, including a balanced diet, regular exercise, and medication, are commonly recommended to manage blood pressure levels. In recent years, research has also highlighted the potential benefits of fish oil and omega-3 fatty acids in reducing high blood pressure.

Omega-3 Fatty Acids and Blood Pressure Regulation:

Omega-3 fatty acids, particularly eicosapentaenoic acid (EPA) and docosahexaenoic acid (DHA), are polyunsaturated fatty acids found abundantly in fatty fish, such as salmon, mackerel, and sardines. These fatty acids play a crucial role in various physiological processes, including the regulation of blood pressure.

Vasodilation and Endothelial Function:

One mechanism through which omega-3 fatty acids may influence blood pressure is by promoting vasodilation and improving endothelial function. The endothelium, the inner lining of blood vessels, plays a vital role in regulating blood flow and blood pressure. Omega-3 fatty acids enhance the production of nitric oxide, a vasodilator, which helps relax blood vessels and improve blood flow, thereby reducing blood pressure.

Anti-inflammatory and Antioxidant Effects:

Chronic inflammation and oxidative stress are associated with the development and progression of hypertension. Omega-3 fatty acids possess anti-inflammatory and antioxidant properties that can mitigate inflammation and oxidative stress, thus potentially reducing blood pressure. By modulating inflammatory markers and reducing oxidative damage, these fatty acids contribute to overall cardiovascular health.

Renin-Angiotensin System Modulation:

The renin-angiotensin system (RAS) plays a very vital role in regulating blood pressure. Omega-3 fatty acids have been shown to modulate the RAS, resulting in decreased production of angiotensin II, a potent vasoconstrictor. By inhibiting angiotensin II synthesis, omega-3 fatty acids promote vasodilation and help lower blood pressure.

Clinical Evidence:
Numerous studies have examined the effects of omega-3 fatty acids on blood pressure in both hypertensive and normotensive individuals. While results have been somewhat mixed, a considerable body of evidence suggests a modest antihypertensive effect of omega-3 fatty acids. Meta-analyses of randomized controlled trials have demonstrated a small but significant reduction in both systolic and diastolic blood pressure with omega-3 supplementation.

Coenzyme Q10

Coenzyme Q10 (CoQ10) is a naturally occurring compound found in the cells of the body, particularly in the mitochondria, which are responsible for producing energy. It plays a crucial role in cellular metabolism and acts as an antioxidant, protecting cells from damage caused by free radicals. CoQ10 has gained attention for its potential benefits in reducing high blood pressure, also known as hypertension.

Research suggests that CoQ10 supplementation may have a positive impact on blood pressure regulation. Here are some ways in which CoQ10 can potentially help reduce high blood pressure:

Antioxidant Activity: *CoQ10 acts as a potent antioxidant, neutralizing harmful free radicals and reducing oxidative stress. Oxidative stress can lead to inflammation and damage to blood vessels, contributing to hypertension. By reducing oxidative stress, CoQ10 may help protect blood vessels and promote healthy cardiovascular function.*

Improved Nitric Oxide Production: *Nitric oxide is a molecule that helps relax and dilate blood vessels, promoting better blood flow and reducing blood pressure. CoQ10 has been found to enhance the production of nitric oxide, leading to improved endothelial function (the inner lining of blood vessels) and vasodilation. This can result in lower blood pressure levels.*

Blood Pressure Regulation: *CoQ10 may help regulate blood pressure by affecting the balance of certain signaling molecules involved in vascular tone and fluid balance. It has been observed to inhibit the production of endothelin-1, a potent vasoconstrictor, while promoting the release of prostacyclin, a vasodilator.*

These actions contribute to the relaxation of blood vessels, leading to lower blood pressure.

Anti-inflammatory Effects: Chronic inflammation is linked to the development of hypertension. CoQ10 has been found to possess anti-inflammatory properties, which can help reduce inflammation in the blood vessels and prevent damage. By modulating inflammatory processes, CoQ10 may contribute to the maintenance of healthy blood pressure levels.

It's important to note that while CoQ10 shows promise in reducing high blood pressure, it should not be considered a standalone treatment for hypertension. It is typically used as a complementary therapy alongside conventional approaches recommended by healthcare professionals. If you have high blood pressure or any other medical condition, it is crucial to consult with your healthcare provider before starting any supplementation regimen.

Remember, individual responses to CoQ10 may vary, and the appropriate dosage should be determined by a healthcare professional based on your specific needs and health status.

Hibiscus Tea

Hibiscus tea, derived from the vibrant flowers of the Hibiscus sabdariffa plant, has been consumed for centuries for its refreshing taste and numerous health benefits. Among its many potential advantages, recent research suggests that hibiscus tea may aid in reducing high blood pressure, a prevalent cardiovascular condition worldwide. This note explores the mechanism behind this effect and highlights the potential benefits of incorporating hibiscus tea into a healthy lifestyle.

The Role of Hibiscus Tea in High Blood Pressure Management:

Blood Pressure Regulation: *Studies have shown that hibiscus tea consumption can lead to a significant decrease in both systolic and diastolic blood pressure levels. This effect may be attributed to the presence of bioactive compounds, such as anthocyanins, flavonoids, and polyphenols, which possess vasodilatory properties. These compounds help relax the blood vessels, promoting better blood flow and reducing pressure on arterial walls.*

Antioxidant Activity: *Hibiscus tea is known for its potent antioxidant properties. Antioxidants help combat oxidative stress, which plays a crucial role in the development and progression of hypertension. By neutralizing free radicals and reducing inflammation,* hibiscus tea may help protect blood vessels from damage and improve overall cardiovascular health.

Diuretic Effect: Hibiscus tea possesses mild diuretic properties, promoting increased urine production and sodium excretion. This action may contribute to blood pressure reduction by reducing fluid volume and sodium levels in the body. By encouraging the elimination of excess fluids, hibiscus tea can help alleviate the strain on the cardiovascular system and aid in blood pressure management.

LDL Cholesterol Reduction: High blood pressure often coexists with elevated levels of LDL (low-density lipoprotein) cholesterol, which contributes to the development of atherosclerosis. Research suggests that hibiscus tea may help lower LDL cholesterol levels, thus potentially reducing the risk of cardiovascular diseases associated with high blood pressure.

Incorporating Hibiscus Tea into a Healthy Lifestyle: To harness the potential benefits of hibiscus tea in reducing high blood pressure, it is essential to adopt a holistic approach to cardiovascular health. Here are some recommendations:

Regular Consumption: Drink hibiscus tea regularly as part of a balanced diet. The tea can be brewed from dried hibiscus petals, which are available in many health food stores.

Lifestyle Modifications: *Complement your tea consumption with other healthy lifestyle habits. Engage in regular physical activity, maintain a balanced diet rich in fruits, vegetables, and whole grains, limit sodium intake, manage stress levels, and avoid smoking and excessive alcohol consumption.*

Consultation with Healthcare Provider: *If you have been diagnosed with hypertension or are taking medications for blood pressure management, consult your healthcare provider before incorporating hibiscus tea into your routine.*

While hibiscus tea is not a substitute for medical treatment, it may be a valuable addition to a comprehensive approach to managing high blood pressure. Its ability to promote blood vessel relaxation, exhibit antioxidant activity, act as a diuretic, and reduce LDL cholesterol levels suggests potential benefits for cardiovascular health. As with any dietary change, it is important to consult with a healthcare professional before making significant modifications to your routine.

Flaxseed

Flaxseed, also known as linseed, is a nutrient-rich plant-based food that has gained recognition for its potential health benefits. Among its various properties, flaxseed has shown promise in helping to reduce high blood pressure, also known as hypertension. Here's a short note on how flaxseed can contribute to managing hypertension:

Omega-3 Fatty Acids: *Flaxseed is an excellent source of alpha-linolenic acid (ALA), which is an omega-3 fatty acid. Omega-3 fatty acids are known for their beneficial effects on cardiovascular health, including lowering blood pressure. ALA has been found to help reduce inflammation and improve the function of blood vessels, which can contribute to lowering blood pressure levels.*

Fiber Content: *Flaxseed is very rich in dietary fiber, both soluble and insoluble. The soluble fiber in flaxseed, particularly mucilage, has been associated with blood pressure-lowering effects. Soluble fiber helps regulate blood sugar levels and cholesterol levels, which can indirectly contribute to managing hypertension.*

Lignans: *Flaxseed have lignans, which are phytoestrogens with antioxidant properties. These lignans have been found to have a positive impact on cardiovascular health, including blood pressure regulation. They may help relax blood vessels and improve blood flow, which can help lower blood pressure.*

Nitric Oxide Production: *Flaxseed has shown the ability to increase the production of nitric oxide in the* body. Nitric oxide acts as a vasodilator, meaning it helps widen blood vessels and improve blood flow. By enhancing nitric oxide production, flaxseed can aid in reducing high blood pressure.

It's important to note that while flaxseed can be a beneficial addition to a healthy diet, it should not replace prescribed medications or professional medical advice for managing high blood pressure.

Beetroot Juice

Uncontrolled hypertension can increase the risk of heart disease, stroke, and other complications. While there are various approaches to managing blood pressure, one natural remedy that has gained attention is beetroot juice. This note explores how beetroot juice can help reduce high blood pressure and improve overall cardiovascular health.

Nitric Oxide Production:
Beetroot juice contains a lot of nitrates, which are converted into nitric oxide in the body. Nitric oxide plays the role of a vasodilator, meaning it helps widen and relax blood vessels. By dilating blood vessels, nitric oxide improves blood flow and reduces resistance, thus lowering blood pressure levels. The increase in nitric oxide production from consuming beetroot juice can have a positive impact on hypertensive individuals.

Lowered Peripheral Resistance:
Peripheral resistance refers to the force exerted by blood vessels against the flow of blood. High peripheral resistance is a common characteristic of hypertension. The nitrates present in beetroot juice have been found to reduce peripheral resistance, making it easier for blood to flow through the vessels. This effect can result in a decrease in blood pressure readings over time.

Antioxidant Properties:
Beetroot juice is packed with antioxidants, particularly betalains and polyphenols. These compounds help neutralize harmful free radicals that are in the body, and it helps to reduce oxidative stress and inflammation. Oxidative stress can damage blood vessels and contribute to hypertension. By combating oxidative stress, beetroot juice promotes cardiovascular health and may contribute to lowering blood pressure.

Improved Endothelial Function:
The endothelium is the inside lining of the blood vessels. Dysfunction of the endothelium can impair blood vessel dilation and contribute to high blood pressure. Beetroot juice has been found to enhance endothelial function by improving nitric oxide availability and reducing inflammation. By supporting healthy endothelial function, beetroot juice can play a role in reducing high blood pressure.

Dosage and Precautions:

While beetroot juice offers potential benefits for individuals with high blood pressure, it is essential to exercise caution and consult with a healthcare professional. The optimal dosage varies depending on factors such as individual health, existing conditions, and medication use. Additionally, beetroot juice may cause temporary discoloration of urine and stool due to its pigments, which is harmless.

Beetroot juice can be a valuable addition to a comprehensive approach for managing high blood pressure. Its high nitrate content, ability to enhance nitric oxide production, lower peripheral resistance, antioxidant properties, and support for endothelial function collectively contribute to its potential blood pressure-lowering effects.

MANAGING HIGH BLOOD PRESSURE WITH RELAXATION TECHNIQUES

Deep Breathing Exercises

In the hustle and bustle of our fast-paced lives, it's essential to pause and take a moment to prioritize our well-being. One powerful tool that can help us achieve this is deep breathing exercises, which have shown promise in reducing high blood pressure.

Imagine the act of inhaling and exhaling as a symphony of tranquility, sweeping away the stress and tension that can elevate our blood pressure. Deep breathing exercises provide a gentle yet impactful way to tap into the healing power of our breath.

When practiced regularly, deep breathing exercises can have a remarkable impact on our cardiovascular health. By consciously slowing down our breathing, inhaling deeply through the nose and exhaling slowly through the mouth, we stimulate the relaxation response in our bodies. This, in turn, can help lower blood pressure levels over time.

Engaging in deep breathing exercises not only helps to calm our minds and promote a sense of inner peace but also encourages better oxygenation and circulation throughout our bodies. As a result, our blood vessels relax, and the workload on our heart decreases, contributing to a healthier cardiovascular system.

Remember, though, that deep breathing exercises should be seen as a complementary approach to managing high blood pressure. It's important to consult with your healthcare provider and follow their guidance, as they can provide personalized advice based on your unique health circumstances.

So, take a moment each day to embrace the power of deep breathing. Find a peaceful spot, close your eyes, and let your breath become your guiding light. Through the simple act of inhaling and exhaling consciously, you can embark on a journey towards greater well-being and blood pressure control.

Progressive Muscle Relaxation

Progressive Muscle Relaxation (PMR) is a therapeutic technique that involves consciously tensing and relaxing various muscle groups to induce a state of deep relaxation. This method has gained recognition as an effective approach to manage stress and anxiety, and recent studies suggest its potential benefits in reducing high blood pressure. In this note, we will explore how

PMR can aid in lowering blood pressure and provide guidelines on how to practice it.

Reducing High Blood Pressure with PMR:

Stress Reduction: *Chronic stress is a significant contributor to high blood pressure. PMR helps individuals relax their muscles and calms the mind, thereby reducing stress and tension. By engaging in PMR, people can experience a sense of relaxation and tranquility, leading to a decrease in blood pressure levels.*

Muscle Tension Release: *Tense muscles can constrict blood vessels, impeding proper blood flow and potentially elevating blood pressure. Through PMR, individuals systematically tense and release various muscle groups, promoting a state of physical relaxation. This process encourages blood vessels to dilate, facilitating improved blood circulation and contributing to reduced blood pressure.*

Enhanced Mind-Body Connection: *PMR involves focusing on the sensations of tension and relaxation in specific muscle groups. By honing in on these bodily sensations, individuals cultivate a heightened mind-body connection. This increased awareness can help individuals recognize and manage early signs of stress, enabling them to intervene and prevent stress-related blood pressure spikes.*

How to Practice PMR:

Find a Quiet Environment: *Choose a calm and quiet space where you can relax without disturbances.*

Get Comfortable: *Sit or lie down in a comfortable position, ensuring your body is fully supported.*

Start with Deep Breaths: *Take a few slow, deep breaths to center yourself and prepare for the exercise.*

Muscle Group Sequence: *Begin with one muscle group, such as your hands or shoulders. Tense the muscles in that group for 5-10 seconds, then release the tension while focusing on the sensation of relaxation for 15-20 seconds. Proceed to the next muscle group and repeat the process.*

Progress Through the Body: *Continue moving systematically through different muscle groups, such as the arms, chest, abdomen, legs, and feet. Gradually work your way from one group to the next, tensing and releasing each group in turn.*

Practice Regularly: *Aim to practice PMR for 10-20 minutes at least once per day. Consistency is key to experiencing the full benefits of this technique.*

Progressive Muscle Relaxation offers a valuable and accessible strategy for managing high blood pressure. By incorporating PMR into their daily routine, individuals can effectively reduce stress, release muscle tension, and improve their overall mind-body connection.

Biofeedback

Biofeedback is a therapeutic technique that enables individuals to gain awareness and control over their physiological processes. It has shown promising results in managing various conditions, including high blood pressure (hypertension). This note explores how biofeedback can help reduce high blood pressure and discusses some common biofeedback techniques employed for this purpose.

Biofeedback and High Blood Pressure:
Biofeedback utilizes instruments that measure and provide real-time feedback on physiological parameters such as blood pressure, heart rate, and muscle tension. By observing this feedback, individuals can gain insight into their body's responses and learn techniques to self-regulate these processes. Biofeedback training can aid in reducing high blood pressure through the following mechanisms:

Relaxation and Stress Reduction: *Chronic stress and tension contribute to high blood pressure. Biofeedback techniques, such as deep breathing exercises,* *progressive muscle relaxation, and mindfulness meditation, can help individuals achieve a state of relaxation and lower their stress levels. These practices encourage the body to activate its natural relaxation response, leading to a decrease in blood pressure.*

Heart Rate Variability (HRV) Training: *HRV refers to the variation in time intervals between consecutive heartbeats. Higher HRV is normally associated with better cardiovascular health. Biofeedback devices can measure HRV and provide feedback on the heart's rhythm. Through HRV training, individuals can learn to modulate their heart rate patterns, promoting a more balanced autonomic nervous system response and ultimately reducing blood pressure.*

Biofeedback-Assisted Breathing: *Controlled breathing exercises play a crucial role in managing blood pressure. Biofeedback devices can guide individuals in maintaining a specific breathing rate or pattern, such as slow and deep breaths. By synchronizing their breathing with the feedback, individuals can induce a relaxation response, leading to lowered blood pressure.*

Biofeedback Techniques:
Biofeedback for hypertension typically involves the use of devices that monitor blood pressure, heart rate, or HRV. These devices may include electronic sensors, cuffs, or wearable devices. Here are a few commonly used biofeedback techniques for reducing high blood pressure:

Electrodermal Activity (EDA) Biofeedback: *Measures skin conductance, which reflects sympathetic nervous system activity. EDA biofeedback helps individuals identify and regulate their stress responses, thus aiding blood pressure control.*

Thermal Biofeedback: *Utilizes sensors to measure skin temperature changes, primarily in the hands. By increasing hand temperature, individuals can enhance peripheral blood flow, leading to blood pressure reduction.*

Heart Rate Variability (HRV) Biofeedback: *Monitors heart rate patterns and provides real-time feedback. HRV biofeedback training helps individuals improve their autonomic nervous system balance and lower blood pressure.*

Biofeedback offers a non-invasive and empowering approach to managing high blood pressure. By providing individuals with real-time information about their physiological processes, it enables them to develop self-regulation skills, reduce stress, and promote relaxation. Incorporating biofeedback techniques into a comprehensive hypertension treatment plan may contribute to better blood pressure control and improved overall cardiovascular health. It is important to consult healthcare professionals or trained biofeedback practitioners to ensure safe and effective implementation of biofeedback practices.

NATURAL REMEDIES AND PRACTICES

Acupuncture

Acupuncture is an ancient Chinese medical practice that involves stimulating specific points on the body to promote healing and alleviate various health conditions. It is widely used as a complementary therapy for managing high blood pressure or hypertension. While it's important to note that acupuncture should not replace conventional medical treatments for high blood pressure, it may offer additional support and help promote overall well-being.

In acupuncture, fine needles are inserted into specific points on the body, known as acupoints. These acupoints are believed to be connected to pathways called meridians, through which vital energy, or Qi, flows. By stimulating these acupoints, acupuncture aims to restore the balance of Qi and improve the body's overall functioning.

When it comes to reducing high blood pressure, acupuncture focuses on specific acupoints related to cardiovascular health. These points may be located on the wrists, ankles, legs, or ears. The selection of acupoints and the treatment plan are individualized based on the person's unique condition and overall health.

Acupuncture treatments for high blood pressure typically involve multiple sessions. During each session, the acupuncturist inserts the fine needles into the chosen acupoints, which may cause a mild sensation or tingling. The needles are usually left in place for around 20 to 30 minutes while the person rests comfortably. Some practitioners may also incorporate other techniques such as electroacupuncture, which involves a gentle electric current applied to the needles.

The potential mechanisms through which acupuncture may help reduce high blood pressure are not yet fully understood. However, it is believed that acupuncture may have several positive effects on the body, including:

***Promoting relaxation:** Acupuncture may help reduce stress and promote a state of relaxation, which can have a positive impact on blood pressure levels.*

***Modulating the autonomic nervous system:** Acupuncture may influence the autonomic nervous system, which plays a crucial role in regulating blood pressure. By balancing the sympathetic and parasympathetic divisions of the nervous system, acupuncture may help normalize blood pressure.*

Enhancing blood circulation: *Acupuncture may improve blood flow and circulation, which can positively affect blood pressure regulation.*

It's important to remember that acupuncture should be performed by a qualified and licensed acupuncturist. It is recommended to consult with a healthcare professional before starting acupuncture treatments, especially if you have high blood pressure or any underlying medical conditions.

While acupuncture may offer potential benefits for managing high blood pressure, it should not replace lifestyle modifications or prescribed medications. A comprehensive approach that combines acupuncture with a healthy diet, regular exercise, stress management techniques, and appropriate medical treatment can provide the best outcomes for managing high blood pressure.

Aromatherapy

Aromatherapy is a holistic practice that utilizes the natural scents and aromatic properties of essential oils to promote physical and emotional well-being. While it is not a substitute for medical treatment, aromatherapy can be used as a complementary therapy to help reduce high blood pressure, also known as hypertension. Here are some natural remedies and practices in aromatherapy that can potentially aid in managing high blood pressure:

Lavender Essential Oil: *Lavender is renowned for its calming and soothing properties. Inhaling lavender essential oil can help reduce stress and anxiety, which are contributing factors to high blood pressure. Add a few drops of lavender oil to a diffuser or inhale it directly from the bottle to experience its calming effects.*

"Ylang-Ylang" Essential Oil: *"Ylang-ylang" oil is known for its ability to promote relaxation and lower blood pressure. It has a sweet, floral scent that can help reduce stress and induce a sense of calmness. Dilute "ylang-ylang" oil with a carrier oil and apply it to your wrists or temples, or add it to a warm bath for a relaxing soak.*

Bergamot Essential Oil: *Bergamot oil has uplifting and mood-enhancing properties. It can help relieve stress and anxiety, which may contribute to high blood pressure. Use bergamot oil in a diffuser to create a* *refreshing and calming atmosphere, or dilute it with a carrier oil and apply it topically.*

Lemon Essential Oil: *Lemon oil is invigorating and refreshing, and it may help improve circulation and reduce blood pressure. Add a few drops of lemon oil to a diffuser or mix it with a carrier oil for a stimulating massage.*

Aromatherapy Massage: *Massage therapy combined with aromatherapy can be beneficial for reducing stress and promoting relaxation, which in turn may help lower blood pressure. Dilute your chosen essential oil with a carrier oil such as almond or jojoba oil, and use it during a gentle massage. Alternatively, seek the assistance of a trained aromatherapist for a customized massage session.*

Inhalation Techniques: *Inhaling the aroma of essential oils can have immediate effects on the body and mind. You can inhale the scent directly from the bottle, use a diffuser, or create a steam inhalation by adding a few drops of essential oil to a bowl of hot water. Cover your head with a towel and inhale the steam for a few minutes to enjoy the therapeutic benefits.*

Remember, aromatherapy should be used as a complementary therapy and not as a substitute for medical treatment. It is essential to consult with a healthcare professional, such as a doctor or aromatherapist, to determine the appropriate course of action for managing high blood pressure.

Massage Therapy

Massage therapy is a natural and non-invasive approach that can help reduce high blood pressure and promote overall well-being. While it should not replace medical treatment or medication prescribed by a healthcare professional, it can be used as a complementary therapy to support hypertension management. Here are some key natural remedies and practices in massage therapy that can be beneficial:

Relaxation Massage: *A relaxation massage focuses on calming the body and mind, reducing stress and anxiety levels, and promoting a state of relaxation. By inducing relaxation, massage therapy can help lower blood pressure, as stress is a common contributing factor to hypertension.*

Swedish Massage: *Swedish massage techniques involve long, flowing strokes, kneading, and circular movements to increase blood circulation and improve muscle relaxation. Improved blood flow can contribute to lower blood pressure levels over time.*

Aromatherapy Massage: *Aromatherapy involves the use of essential oils to enhance the therapeutic effects of massage. Certain essential oils, such as lavender or chamomile, are known for their calming properties and can help reduce stress and anxiety, thereby potentially lowering blood pressure.*

Deep Tissue Massage: *Deep tissue massage focuses on releasing tension and tightness in deeper layers of muscles and connective tissues. By targeting specific areas of tension, it can help promote relaxation and improve blood flow, potentially contributing to lower blood pressure levels.*

Reflexology: *Reflexology is a technique that involves applying pressure to specific points on the feet or hands that correspond to different organs and systems in the body. Stimulating these reflex points may help improve blood circulation, reduce stress, and support overall relaxation.*

It's important to note that the effectiveness of massage therapy in reducing high blood pressure can vary among individuals. Furthermore, it is crucial to consult with a qualified massage therapist and inform them about your specific health condition, including hypertension, before starting any massage treatment.

In conclusion, massage therapy can be a valuable complementary practice for individuals with high blood pressure. By promoting relaxation, improving blood circulation, and reducing stress levels, it may contribute to managing hypertension. However, it's essential to consult with healthcare professionals and use massage therapy as part of a comprehensive treatment plan for high blood pressure.

Chiropractic Care

Chiropractic care involves non-invasive techniques that aim to optimize the body's natural healing abilities. This note explores how chiropractic care can potentially reduce high blood pressure and provides insights into the practices involved.

Chiropractic Care and High Blood Pressure:
Chiropractic care primarily focuses on the relationship between the spine and the nervous system. Practitioners believe that misalignments or subluxations in the spine can disrupt nerve communication and contribute to various health issues, including high blood pressure. By employing various natural remedies and practices, chiropractors aim to restore proper spinal alignment and enhance overall wellness, which may positively impact blood pressure levels.

Spinal Adjustments:
Spinal adjustments, also known as spinal manipulations, are the core treatment technique used by chiropractors.

Through manual adjustments or specialized instruments, chiropractors apply controlled forces to specific areas of the spine. The goal is to correct misalignments and restore proper joint function. Research suggests that spinal adjustments may have a positive impact on blood pressure by reducing nerve interference and enhancing nervous system function.

Lifestyle Modifications:
Chiropractors often provide guidance on lifestyle modifications that can support overall health and potentially help manage blood pressure. These may include dietary recommendations, exercise routines, stress reduction techniques, and weight management strategies. By addressing these factors, chiropractic care aims to create a holistic approach to blood pressure management.

Stress Reduction:
Chiropractic care incorporates stress reduction techniques that can potentially contribute to lower blood pressure levels. Stress can significantly impact blood pressure, and chiropractors may employ relaxation techniques, such as massage therapy, stretching exercises, or breathing exercises, to help patients reduce stress levels and promote overall well-being.

Complementary Therapies:
Chiropractic care may integrate complementary therapies to further support blood pressure management. These may include acupuncture,

nutritional counseling, herbal supplements, or homeopathic remedies. However, the effectiveness of these approaches for blood pressure management varies, and it's crucial to consult with a qualified chiropractor before considering any additional therapies.

While chiropractic care offers natural remedies and practices that may help reduce high blood pressure, it is important to note that it should not be considered a standalone treatment for hypertension. Chiropractic care can be utilized as a complementary approach alongside traditional medical management and lifestyle modifications. Consultation with a healthcare professional, such as a chiropractor or primary care physician, is essential to determine the most appropriate course of action for managing high blood pressure effectively.

ADDITIONAL CONSIDERATIONS AND PRECAUTIONS

Consultation with Healthcare Professional

Consultation with a healthcare professional is crucial when dealing with high blood pressure, also known as hypertension. High blood pressure is a common and potentially serious condition that affects millions of people all over the world. Seeking guidance from a healthcare professional can provide valuable insights, personalized advice, and appropriate treatment options. Here are a few key reasons why consultation with a healthcare professional is important when managing high blood pressure:

Accurate Diagnosis: *Consulting a healthcare professional allows for an accurate diagnosis of high blood pressure. They will measure your blood pressure using a blood pressure cuff and evaluate your overall health condition. This helps determine the severity of your condition and whether any underlying causes or risk factors are contributing to it.*

Individualized Treatment Plan: *Healthcare professionals can develop a tailored treatment plan based on your specific health needs and circumstances.*

They will consider factors such as your blood pressure readings, overall health, age, medical history, and other existing conditions. This personalized approach ensures that the treatment plan is effective and safe for you.

Lifestyle Modifications: *Managing high blood pressure often involves making certain lifestyle changes. A healthcare professional can provide guidance on adopting a healthy diet, reducing sodium intake, incorporating regular physical activity, managing stress, and quitting smoking. These modifications can significantly contribute to controlling blood pressure levels and improving overall health.*

Medication Management: *In some cases, medication may be necessary to control high blood pressure. Healthcare professionals are knowledgeable about the different types of antihypertensive medications available and can prescribe the most appropriate one based on your condition. They will monitor your response to the medication, adjust the dosage if needed, and manage any potential side effects.*

Regular Monitoring: *High blood pressure requires ongoing monitoring to ensure it is effectively managed and does not lead to complications. A healthcare professional will schedule follow-up appointments to assess your blood pressure, review your progress, and make any necessary adjustments to your treatment plan. Regular monitoring helps to identify any changes or issues promptly.*

Education and Support: *Consulting with a healthcare professional provides an opportunity to learn more about high blood pressure, its causes, potential risks, and ways to prevent complications. They can answer your questions, address concerns, and provide valuable educational resources. This support and knowledge empower you to take an active role in managing your blood pressure effectively.*

Remember, high blood pressure is a chronic condition that requires ongoing attention and management. Regular consultations with a healthcare professional play a vital role in controlling your blood pressure levels, reducing associated risks, and improving your overall well-being.

Combining Natural Remedies With Medications

High blood pressure is a serious health concern that, if left uncontrolled, can lead to various complications such as heart disease, stroke, and kidney problems. While prescription medications are often prescribed to manage high blood pressure effectively, some individuals may be interested in complementing their treatment with natural remedies. Here are a few points to consider when combining natural remedies with medications to reduce high blood pressure:

Consultation with a healthcare professional: *Before incorporating any natural remedies into your treatment plan, it is crucial to consult with your healthcare provider. They can assess your medical history, current medications, and individual health needs to determine the suitability of combining natural remedies with prescribed drugs. This step is important to ensure there are no potential interactions or contraindications that may impact your health.*

Awareness of potential interactions: *Natural remedies, such as herbal supplements, can interact with certain medications, including those used to manage high blood pressure. For example, some herbal supplements like St. John's wort, ginkgo biloba, and garlic may interfere with blood pressure medications or increase the risk of bleeding. It is vital to be aware of these potential interactions and discuss them with your healthcare provider to make informed decisions.*

Complementary approaches: *Natural remedies should be viewed as complementary to prescribed medications rather than replacements. They may provide additional support in managing high blood pressure, but they should not be relied upon as standalone treatments. Medications prescribed by your doctor have undergone rigorous testing and research to prove their* effectiveness in controlling blood pressure, and they should be the primary focus of your treatment plan.

Lifestyle modifications: Alongside natural remedies and medications, adopting a healthy lifestyle can greatly contribute to managing high blood pressure. This includes maintaining a balanced diet rich in fruits, vegetables, whole grains, and lean proteins, limiting salt intake, engaging in regular physical activity, managing stress levels, and avoiding smoking and excessive alcohol consumption. These lifestyle modifications, combined with medication and natural remedies, can have a positive impact on blood pressure control.

Natural remedies with potential benefits: While evidence supporting the effectiveness of natural remedies in reducing high blood pressure is limited, some substances have shown promising results in preliminary studies. For example, coenzyme Q10 (CoQ10), omega-3 fatty acids, hibiscus tea, and beetroot juice have been suggested to have modest blood pressure-lowering effects. However, it is important to note that more extensive research is needed to establish their efficacy and safety profiles.

 Combining natural remedies with prescribed medications to reduce high blood pressure can be considered as long as it is done under the guidance of a healthcare professional. The consultation will help ensure there are no potential interactions or contraindications, and that the primary focus remains on *the prescribed medication. Additionally, incorporating a healthy lifestyle, including dietary changes and regular exercise, is essential for overall blood pressure management. It is important to remember that natural remedies should not replace prescribed medications, but rather be viewed as supplementary tools to support blood pressure control.*

Regular Blood Pressure Monitoring

Regular blood pressure monitoring is a vital aspect of maintaining overall health and preventing potential complications related to hypertension. Hypertension is the force exerted by circulating blood on the walls of blood vessels . It is measured in millimeters of mercury (mmHg) and is typically represented by two values: systolic pressure over diastolic pressure.

Regular blood pressure monitoring involves measuring and recording blood pressure readings at regular intervals. This can be done at home using a home blood pressure monitor or by visiting a healthcare professional. Here are a few key points to consider regarding regular blood pressure monitoring:

Early Detection of Hypertension: *Regular monitoring helps identify high blood pressure (hypertension) early on, as it often presents with no obvious symptoms. Hypertension is a significant risk factor for various health conditions, including heart disease, stroke, kidney disease, and more. By detecting hypertension early,* appropriate measures can be taken to manage and control blood pressure effectively.

Treatment Effectiveness: For individuals already diagnosed with hypertension, regular blood pressure monitoring provides essential feedback on the effectiveness of their treatment plan. It helps determine if lifestyle modifications or medication adjustments are necessary to achieve target blood pressure levels.

Personalized Blood Pressure Targets: Regular monitoring allows healthcare providers to establish personalized blood pressure targets based on an individual's age, overall health, and risk factors. Maintaining blood pressure within the recommended range helps reduce the risk of associated health problems.

Lifestyle Modifications: Monitoring blood pressure regularly encourages individuals to adopt and maintain a healthy lifestyle. It promotes habits such as regular physical activity, a balanced diet, weight management, limited sodium intake, moderation in alcohol consumption, stress reduction, and quitting smoking. These lifestyle changes can significantly contribute to maintaining optimal blood pressure levels.

Awareness and Empowerment: By actively monitoring blood pressure, individuals become more aware of their cardiovascular health and gain a sense of empowerment in managing their well-being. It fosters a *proactive approach towards health and motivates individuals to take charge of their lifestyle choices.*

Regular blood pressure monitoring is crucial for maintaining cardiovascular health. Whether it is for early detection, treatment evaluation, or promoting a healthy lifestyle, monitoring blood pressure at regular intervals empowers individuals to make informed decisions and take appropriate steps towards achieving and maintaining optimal blood pressure levels.

Potential Side Effects and Allergies

When considering natural remedies to address high blood pressure, it's important to be aware that even though they are generally considered safe, they may still have potential side effects and can cause allergic reactions in some individuals. Here's a brief note on potential side effects and allergies related to natural remedies for high blood pressure:

Hawthorn: *Hawthorn is a herb often used to support cardiovascular health and lower blood pressure. Although it is generally well-tolerated, some individuals may experience digestive upset, headache, dizziness, or palpitations. Allergic reactions to hawthorn are rare but possible, especially in individuals allergic to related plants such as roses or apples.*

Garlic: *Garlic has been recognized for its potential to lower blood pressure. However, excessive consumption or high doses of garlic supplements may cause digestive issues, heartburn, bloating, or allergic reactions in some people. Allergy to garlic is relatively uncommon but can occur, leading to symptoms like skin rash, itching, or respiratory distress.*

Hibiscus: *Hibiscus tea is known for its potential blood pressure-lowering effects. While generally safe, some individuals may experience an upset stomach, gas, or a mild laxative effect. People with known allergies to hibiscus or related plants, such as marshmallow or rose, should exercise caution and monitor for allergic reactions.*

Fish Oil: *Fish oil, which contains omega-3 fatty acids, is commonly used to support heart health. High doses or poor-quality fish oil supplements may lead to side effects like fishy aftertaste, burping, indigestion, or diarrhea. Individuals allergic to fish should avoid fish oil supplements or seek alternative sources of omega-3 fatty acids like algae-based supplements.*

Coenzyme Q10 (CoQ10): *CoQ10 is an antioxidant that plays a role in cardiovascular health. While generally well-tolerated, it can sometimes cause mild side effects such as digestive upset, nausea, or headache. Allergic reactions to CoQ10 are rare but possible, and individuals with known allergies to CoQ10 should avoid its use.*

It's important to note that these are general observations, and individual reactions may vary. If you're considering natural remedies for high blood pressure, it's recommended to consult with a healthcare professional, especially if you have pre-existing medical conditions, take other medications, or have a history of allergies. They can provide personalized guidance and help you make informed decisions regarding natural remedies and their potential side effects.

CONCLUSION

Harmony Within: Holistic Approaches to Lowering High Blood Pressure Naturally" offers a comprehensive and insightful exploration of alternative methods to manage and reduce high blood pressure. Throughout the book, the author skillfully combines scientific evidence with holistic approaches, providing readers with a well-rounded understanding of the subject.

One of the key strengths of this book is its emphasis on addressing high blood pressure through natural and holistic means. Rather than relying solely on medication, the author encourages readers to explore various lifestyle modifications, including exercise, diet, stress management, and alternative therapies. By presenting a wide range of approaches, the book empowers individuals to take an active role in their own health and well-being.

The author's writing style is accessible and engaging, making complex medical concepts easy to understand for readers of all backgrounds. Furthermore, the inclusion of personal stories and case studies adds a human element, making the book relatable and inspiring. Readers will find themselves motivated and encouraged to implement the suggested strategies and techniques.

Additionally, the book places a strong emphasis on the interconnectedness of mind, body, and spirit. It highlights the importance of addressing the underlying emotional and psychological factors that contribute to high blood pressure. By incorporating practices such as meditation, mindfulness, and relaxation techniques, the author encourages readers to achieve a state of balance and harmony within themselves.

While "Harmony Within" offers valuable insights and practical advice, it is important to note that individual results may vary. High blood pressure is a complex condition that often requires a multifaceted approach, including professional medical guidance. Readers should consult with their healthcare providers before making any significant changes to their treatment plans.

Overall, "Harmony Within: Holistic Approaches to Lowering High Blood Pressure Naturally" serves as a valuable resource for individuals seeking alternative ways to manage their high blood pressure. By combining scientific knowledge with holistic practices, the book empowers readers to take control of their health and embark on a journey toward better well-being. It is a testament to the power of holistic approaches in promoting a healthier lifestyle and achieving harmony within oneself.